Immunisation Options

A Simple Guide for Parents Who Care

Dr Isaac Golden

Immunisation Options: A Simple Guide for Parents Who Care
Dr Isaac Golden PhD, DHom, ND, BEc (Hon)
Principal, Aurum Healing Centre
Director, Australasian College of Hahnemannian Homeopathy
Director, Homeopathy International Online College
Honorary Research Fellow. School of Science and Technology.
Federation University Australia.
Head of School and Business Manager Academic, Endeavour College
of Natural Health, 2008-2012
Homeopathic Coordinator, Melbourne College of Natural Medicine,
1995-2004
President, Australian Homeopathic Association (Victoria), 1992-1998
Australian Homeopathic Association, Distinguished Service Award,
13.3.1999

Inquiries:	Postal:	P.O. Box 695, Gisborne, Victoria, 3437,
Australia.	Phone:	+ 61(03) 5427 0880
	e-Mail:	admin@homstudy.net

Web Pages: www.homstudy.net
- link to publications, education or immunisation.

Disclaimer: This book is not intended to replace the services of a qualified practitioner. Any application of the recommendations set forth in the following pages is at the reader's discretion and sole risk.

ISBN-13: 978-1508741992
ISBN-10: 1508741999

Other Publications by the Author:

The Complete Practitioners Manual of Homoeoprophylaxis.
2012.   ISBN-13: 978-1478388050 ISBN-10: 1478388056

Vaccination & Homœoprophylaxis? - A Review of Risks and Alternatives. 7th ed. 2010.   ISBN 978-9578726-7-7

Vaccine Damaged Children: Treatment, Prevention, Reasons. 2010 reprint.   ISBN 978-9578726-6-0

Homœoprophylaxis – A Fifteen Year Clinical Study. 2004.
          ISBN 0-9578-7263-1

Homœoprophylaxis - A Practical and Philosophical Review. 4th ed. 2007.   ISBN 0-646-19529-8

Homœoprophylaxis – A Ten Year Clinical Study. 1997.
          ISBN 0-646-32054-8

Australian Homeopathic Home Prescriber - Part 1. 3rd ed. 2007.
          ISBN 0-646-15057-X

Australian Homeopathic Home Prescriber - Part 2. 2001
          ISBN 0-9578726-0-7

Australian Homeopathic Home Prescriber – Part 3. 2007.
          ISBN 0-9578726-5-3

Homeopathic Treatment of the Energy Bodies. 2002.
          ISBN 0-9578726-1-5

Homeopathic Body-System Prescribing - A Practical Workbook of Sector Remedies, 2nd ed. 2002.   ISBN 0-646-27292-6

OUTLINE

Introduction

There are many difficult conversations in healthcare – how to best assist people dying in pain; policies regarding foetal termination; the ethics of spending a million dollars on a procedure to help one person rather than using that money to assist hundreds of others; and so on. But the conversation that attracts the most venomous disagreement relates to something where all sides have already agreed on the final goal – the maximisation of health of all community members, especially children.

The decision of whether to vaccinate against potentially serious diseases is one of the most difficult that many thousands of parents will face when raising their children. Most allow the decision to be made for them, and vaccinate according to Government recommendations. But a growing number of parents question whether vaccination is the best option for their child based on their assessment of potential benefits and risks.

Given the overwhelming level of vaccination compliance (92% in Australia), one must ask why there is any doubt about this issue at all. The answer for many, including some parents who do vaccinate, is that they have lost trust in orthodox advice. There are real reasons why this has happened, reasons which Health Department literature and pro-vaccination documentaries[1] have all failed to address.

There are tens of thousands of parents in Australia, and countless more internationally, who have witnessed what they believe is damage caused to their children by vaccines. Yet their genuine concerns regarding this link are typically dismissed by orthodox clinicians as being "just coincidence", "hysteria", "ignorance", and so on. These parents live with the consequences of vaccine damage every day of their lives, and believe that such conclusions are arrogant, and dismissive of their genuine concerns.

They are told that vaccines are proven to be safe, yet parents see the huge payouts made in vaccine damage compensation schemes in other countries (America has now passed the $2.8billion mark[2]) proving that some adverse events do occur. They look up Government sites like the VAERS database of adverse events containing hundreds of thousands of entries[3], so they know that there is too much here to be simple "coincidence".

Some questions that need answers

The more informed ask a simple question – *where are the long-term studies examining the holistic health (intellectual, emotional and physical) of age-appropriate, fully vaccinated and completely unvaccinated children?* They don't find such studies. Instead they find a relatively few studies which claim to prove the long-term safety of vaccination, but either they don't consider the holistic health of participants, or don't look at age-appropriate cohorts, or don't compare fully vaccinated and unvaccinated cohorts - the combination of which is necessary to prove long-term safety. And even the studies cited are imperfect – for example, the very large "Danish studies" published in 2002 and 2003, credited with proving that autism is not related to thimerosal and MMR, are weakened by significant confounders and researcher fraud (see Chapter 2 for more details).

So based on careful research, some intelligent and reasonable people ask a second question – *we are told repeatedly that the risks from vaccines are less than the risks from the diseases they prevent, but if the long-term risks are not fully quantified, how can such a statement be scientifically credible?* That question is generally answered by referring to toxicological reports, and the less than adequate long-term studies noted above. For many parents the answer is unsatisfactory.

Finally, some of these parents continue their research and find that there is a middle path – immunising their child homeopathically, a practice which was first used in 1798 (vaccines were first used in 1796).

They are told by orthodox authorities that homeopathically prepared substances have nothing in them so they can't work, and also that there is no evidence of effectiveness. All agree that "nothing" cannot be toxic, so the real question then becomes – is there evidence of effectiveness?

Hands-on Evidence

It is here that I must describe my personal experience involving the collection of evidence. This experience shows that any statement that "there is no evidence" is simply a denial of reality. Of course the evidence may be contested and the results argued over, but existence of evidence supporting claims regarding the effectiveness of homeopathic immunisation is undeniable.

I was first invited to visit Cuba in December 2008 to present at an international conference hosted by the Finlay Institute, which is a W.H.O. accredited vaccine manufacturer. The Cubans described their use of homeopathic immunisation, also called *homoeoprophylaxis* (HP), to control an outbreak of leptospirosis (a potentially fatal, water-born bacterial disease) in 2007 among the residents of the three eastern provinces which were most severely damaged by a severe hurricane – over 2.2 million people. 2008 was an even worse year involving three hurricanes, and the country's food production was only just recovering at the time of the conference. The HP program had been repeated in 2008, but data was not available at the conference regarding that intervention.

I revisited Cuba in 2010, 2012 and 2014, each time to work with the leader of the HP interventions, Dr Gustavo Bracho to analyse the data available. Dr Bracho is not a homeopath; he is a published and an internationally recognised expert in the manufacture of vaccine adjuvants. He worked in Australia at Flinders University during 2004 with a team trying to develop an anti-malarial vaccine.

In 2012 we accessed the raw leptospirosis surveillance data, comprising weekly reports from 15 provinces over 9 years (2000 to 2008) reporting 21 variables. This yielded a matrix with 147,420 possible entries. This included data concerning possible confounders, such as vaccination and chemoprophylaxis, which allowed a careful examination of possible distorting effects. With the permission of the Cubans, I brought this data back to Australia to be examined by mathematicians at an Australian university to determine what other information could be extracted.

The 2008 result was remarkable, and could only be explained by the effectiveness of the HP intervention. Whilst the three hurricanes caused immense damage throughout the country it was again worse in the east, yet the three homeopathically immunised provinces experienced a negligible increase in cases whilst the rest of the country showed significant increases until the dry season in January 2009.

In 2014 we examined data relating to interventions from 2004 to 2014 against Dengue Fever, Cholera, Hepatitis A, Swine Flu and Pneumococcal disease. Unambiguously positive results were obtained[4]. Clearly, any claim that there is no objective data supporting claims regarding the effectiveness of HP are untrue.

The 2008 leptospirosis intervention is but one example - there are many more. It is cited to show that there is significant data available, and that many HP interventions have been conducted, as in the Cuban case, by orthodox scientists and doctors. Many people internationally now know this, so once again claims by orthodox authorities that there is no evidence merely serve to show that either the authorities are making uninformed/unscientific statements, or that they are aware but are intentionally withholding information. Either way, public confidence is destroyed and this leads to groups of people questioning what they are told.

Towards agreement

It is contended that what now seems to be an endless and repetitive battle between pro and anti-vaccination groups would be unnecessary if the Government made three decisions:

1. Ensure that the parents of vaccine-damaged children and the children themselves are appropriately supported, and that these people and other parents genuinely concerned about the possibility of vaccine damage are not attacked as being irresponsible and a danger to the community.

2. Support those parents who would otherwise not vaccinate their children to use homeopathic immunisation. This in turn would lead to an increase in herd immunity. It would also allow coverage against diseases such as malaria, and dengue fever for which there are no vaccines. It would not require Government endorsement of the method, just appropriate paperwork to identify which type of immunisation was being used – vaccination or HP.

3. Establish a Government sponsored study of long-term vaccine safety examining the holist health of age-appropriate, fully vaccinated and unvaccinated children, and publish the full results whatever they might be. They could be compared with similar data studying children who use HP.

I would also suggest that given the legislative protection and Government financial support provided to multinational vaccine manufacturers in most countries, that our Governments evaluate the possibility of having vaccines used in a country be made in the country by a not-for-profit manufacturer. If a small country like Cuba can do this, then so can affluent countries like Australia. A huge country like China could certainly become independent of Big Pharma if they chose. We should not have to bear the costs of a near-mandatory medical procedure (both the direct costs of vaccines themselves as well as the costs of caring for vaccine damaged children and adults), without sharing the financial rewards from making and selling the pharmaceuticals, but this is the existing situation with vaccination.

This divisive issue has caused many societies to become less tolerant places, where free-speech is prevented through selective media bans and the discussion of ideas and options is attacked by academics and scientists who should be the champions of open and objective dialogue. We need to return to evidence – not just selected and convenient results but all the evidence from all sides of this issue. The orthodox response is that all the evidence has been considered and there is no more to discuss. But too many people know that this is not true, and until a fully open conversation is held this issue will never be resolved. And it needs to be – in the best interest of us all.

The Influence of Big Phama

There may be only a few countries in the world where an open conversation can still happen, which is a demonstration of the financial and political influence which multinational pharmaceutical companies (Big Pharma) exert over all aspects of the orthodox health system. This influence was recently examined by Professor J Ioannidis and colleagues, as was found to be utterly pervasive[5].

The finding was reinforced by Lab Fellows from the Edmond J. Safra Center for Ethics at Harvard University who undertook exhaustive research over five years, the findings of which were presented in a series of sixteen articles in the *Journal of Law, Medicine and Ethics*, Vol. 41, No. 3 (2013). They reported that (i) "widespread practices in the medical and pharmaceutical industries can lead to doctors who are psychologically, financially, or intellectually dependent on drug companies, a phenomenon which has resulted in insufficiently tested drugs, many of which cause harmful side effects", (ii) "top medical researchers can be financially tied to drug firms", (iii) "pharmaceutical marketing ... distorts medical practice", (iv) "drug firms are ... funding social network websites for doctors in order to quietly track their opinions on issues that affect their bottom lines", and (v) "lawmakers and patient advocacy organisations can be dependent on money from drug companies, resulting in representation that serves the interests of Big Pharma rather than the public"[6].

The evidence from impeachable orthodox sources shows that the largest multinational pharmaceutical companies (Big Pharma) are corporate criminals. They are regularly convicted and fined billions of dollars in penalties[7]. But their immense wealth means these huge fines are effortlessly absorbed as a cost of doing business. This will not change until Board members and CEOs are held personally liable and jail penalties are imposed.

The actions of these companies have repeatedly demonstrated that they regard patient welfare as unimportant, and a rush for even more profit and higher executive salaries is what dominates their actions. Their corrupting influence has tainted the entire evidence base of pharmaceutical medicine, contaminated the training of medical practitioners, and has seduced politicians into voting for even greater expenditure of public money on pharmaceutical drugs and vaccines.

This means that parents need to be vigilant, to be discerning, to question even the most respectable health authorities, and be prepared to be self-reliant in terms of researching their best health options.

Orthodox medicine has produced wonderful advances in many areas, especially in emergency medicine. It has failed in producing greatly improved long-term holistic health (which is not measured by life-expectancy, but by quality of life). Most doctors working with patients are concerned people who genuinely care for their patients. But they work within a disease-management system which is controlled by Big Pharma. This fact influences much of what follows.

Chapter 1: Decisions for Parents

Figure 1 shows a simple decision-making tree that parents can use. The key questions to answer are:

1. *Which diseases should I target for prevention?* Some diseases are more potentially dangerous than others. Different countries will have different disease risk-profiles, so prevention programs should take into account the potential severity of what is active in each community.
2. *Should I use general prevention or disease-specific prevention?* Making a child as healthy as possible is always advisable, but evidence shows that prevention is maximised when targeted diseases are prevented using disease-specific methods.
3. *Which method of disease-specific prevention should I use – vaccination or homeopathic immunisation (HP)?* The answer generally depends on answers to two further questions;
    (i) What is the long-term safety of vaccination? This is discussed in Chapter 2, and   (ii) What is the effectiveness of homeopathic immunisation? This is discussed in Chapter 3.

Figure 1: A Simple Decision Making Path for Parents

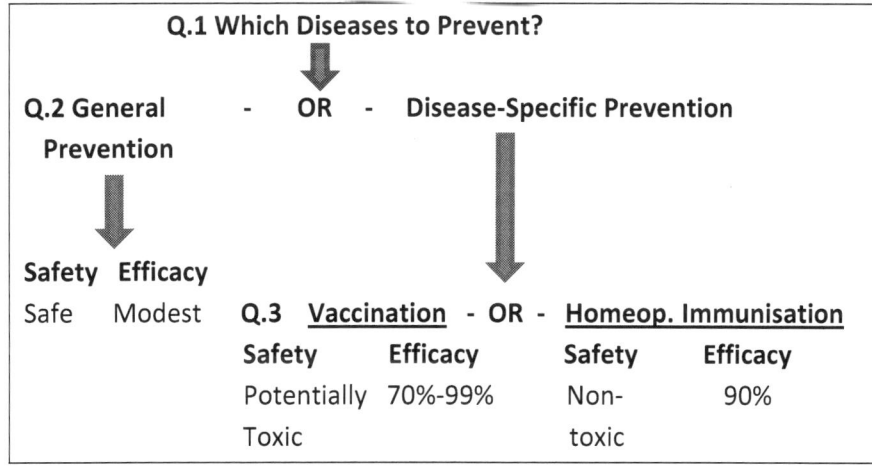

Chapter 2: The Long-Term Safety of Vaccines.

Vaccination has saved many lives since its introduction in 1796. We also know that it has cost lives, and has caused a range of immediate distress in recipients from minor discomfort at the injection site to brain damage (as shown below). What is less certain is the long-term safety of vaccination. The following six aspects of safety will be examined.

1.   Evidence from official vaccine damage compensation schemes.
2.   Official non-science statements about vaccine safety.
3.   The failure to evaluate the impact of total vaccine load.
4.   The failure to compare vaccinated with completely unvaccinated children.
5.   Large studies that don't prove what they claim to prove.
6.   The possible link between infant mortality rates and vaccination.

Note that some material following can be technical, but it is important to know the facts so that you can be well informed when talking to people who hold different opinions.

1.   Vaccines can cause significant damage to recipients, as evidenced by compensation for vaccine damage paid by some Governments. For example, in the United States since the first Vaccine Injury Compensation claims were made in 1989, through to 2014, 3,535 compensation payments have been made, $2,671,223,269.97 disbursed to petitioners and $109,305,515.01 paid to cover attorney's fees and other legal costs[8]. Governments such as the United Kingdom and Japan have also paid out hundreds of millions of dollars in vaccine damage compensation. Australia and Canada are the only developed western countries who do not have vaccine damage compensation schemes.

2.   Official publications make claims such as; "Vaccines, like other medicines, can have side effects", but that "The great majority of side-effects that follow vaccination are minor and short lived" and that "all vaccines in use in Australia provide benefits that greatly outweigh their

risks"[9]. Apart from the fact that it seems highly unlikely that billions of dollars would have been paid in vaccine damage compensation if this statement were totally accurate, the fact remains that the long-term safety of vaccines has been poorly studied as evidenced by the following material, so such statements are not based in science.

3.   No studies have compared the total impact on health of all 28 doses of different vaccines given to children by 4 years of age with completely unvaccinated children. The closest we have is a study where macaque monkeys were given the full vaccination schedule and others not, and the impact on their brains studied using sophisticated brain imaging. This study found that "maturational changes in amygdala volume and binding capacity of ["C]DPN in the amygdala was significantly altered in infant macaques receiving the vaccine schedule. The macaque infant is a relevant animal model in which to investigate specific environmental exposures and structural/functional neuroimaging during neurodevelopment", i.e. **the amygdala's in the vaccinated primates were significantly affected leading to autistic type behaviour**[10].

4.   No substantial studies have been published examining the holistic impact of vaccines, i.e. the effect on the intellectual, emotional and physical development of fully vaccinated and totally unvaccinated groups of age-appropriate children. Four small studies that attempted to do this all found that vaccinated children were much less healthy than unvaccinated children[11],[12],[13],[14].

5.   Large, long-term studies which claim that vaccines do not cause specific adverse effects (such as autism, epilepsy etc) are methodologically dubious, leading to questionable conclusions. And official statements keep re-quoting these same few studies. For example, the 2012 publication by the Australian Academy of Science (AAS), *The Science of Immunisation: Questions and Answers*, a current official Australian document supporting vaccination, asks the question "Does

the MMR vaccine cause autism?" In concluding that it does not, they quote two frequently referenced publications as evidence[15].

(a) Firstly, the AAS say that "Many comprehensive studies subsequently ruled out this suggested link by showing conclusively that rates of autism are the same in children who have and have not been vaccinated", quoting the Institute of Medicine[16]. In fact in Chapter 4 of the 2012 IOM report, where they examine the possible association between autism and the MMR vaccine, shows that they rely on four studies which they said "were judged to have negligible limitations; all reported null associations (on average) between MMR vaccination and subsequent autism diagnosis (or onset) and the overall precision was high" (page 148).

However one of the studies using a large retrospective cohort from Denmark is far from having negligible limitations. Three obvious confounders have been identified; (i) changed accounting methods in 1995 incorporating outpatient with inpatient visits; (ii) change in 1994 of autism diagnosis criteria from ICD8 to ICD10; (iii) failure to account for the inclusion of a large outpatient clinic in 1992 which accounted for 20% of all cases.

In addition, these 4 studies did not compare fully vaccinated and totally unvaccinated infants; they compared infants who had been vaccinated including with MMR and those who had been vaccinated but not with MMR. Clearly these are not children who have "not been vaccinated" as claimed by AAS.

(b) Secondly, the AAS state that "any link between thimerosal, which was previously used in minute quantities in vaccines, and autism has also been excluded", quoting a 2004 study by Parker et al[17]. In fact, these authors rejected 3 cohort studies showing a positive association and supported 4 that rejected an association between ASD and vaccination. However they acknowledged that "In a cohort study that finds no association, it is important to assess the study's power to detect a significant association, if it existed; none of the four quality cohort publications did so", and that "there may be a small chance that a clinically important association could not be detected by an individual study" (page 802).

Apart from the fact that some Australian vaccines still do contain thimerosal, it can be seen that the evidence is suggestive, not conclusive. The AAS did not look critically at the 4 studies on which their conclusion was based. One of the 4 is the follow-up Danish study affected by the confounders noted above. An analysis removing these confounders resulted in the 2003 study data revealing a significant reduction in autism cases when thimerosal was removed from vaccines rather than the opposite conclusion drawn in the paper[18].

One of two authors in both Danish reports, Dr Poul Thorsen, has been accused of fraud by Danish police, and emails obtained under freedom of information laws show that he and other authors withheld data from inclusion in the 2003 study that would have led to an opposite finding, viz. "the incidence and prevalence (of autism) are still decreasing in 2001"[19].

So it is clear that the data on which major claims of vaccine safety rest are questionable. The research which would settle this matter once and for all has never been undertaken, OR, if it has then it has never been published.

6.   A statistically significant association exists between the number of vaccines given and a nations' infant mortality rate[20]. "Linear regression analysis of unweighted mean IMRs showed a high statistically significant correlation between increasing number of vaccine doses and increasing infant mortality rates, with r=0.992 (p=0.0009)". Association does not prove causation, but there is a situation here to be answered not avoided, as is happening.

These six points show that there is a real case to answer regarding long-term vaccine safety. There are a few large, long-term studies that are repeatedly quoted in official Government publications used to demonstrate that vaccines are safe in the long-term. These studies are flawed. They do **not** conclusively prove that vaccines are safe in the long-term.

One test which parents can apply is to ask whether the doctor wishing to administer vaccines to their child is prepared to provide them with a written **personal** guarantee that their child will not be harmed by the vaccines, and that if the child is harmed that the doctor will assume full financial responsibility for remedying the vaccine damage. If not, then the doctor must acknowledge that the parents have genuine grounds for concern.

Chapter 3: The Effectiveness of Homoeopathic Immunisation (HP)

"Official" publications claim that there is no evidence supporting the effectiveness of HP. These claims are unscientific because they simply ignore the substantial evidence that is available. Disagreement with the findings derived from the evidence is a different discussion to saying that evidence does not exist.

An examination of the considerable clinical history of homeopathy, of articles published in peer-reviewed homeopathic and other journals, as well as in books and proceedings of medical conferences shows that there are now four types of evidence which support the effectiveness of HP:

1. Over 200 years of recorded clinical effectiveness spread throughout the homoeopathic literature in many languages (HP was first used in 1798, vaccines first used in 1796). Most of this clinical evidence was recorded by homoeopaths who were also doctors of medicine. This information is useful, but does not yield measures of effectiveness.

2. A number of short-term interventions of HP have been published in English. The most impressive is a 1998 intervention which involved 65,826 children using the homoeopathic preventative against meningococcal disease (type B), with an unimmunised control group of 23,539 children, showing an efficacy of 95% after 6 months and 91% after 12 months[21]. Other smaller interventions in a wide range of diseases produced a consistent level of effectiveness around 90%.

3. I conducted a study of the effectiveness of long-term HP from 1985 to 2004, and which formed one part of my PhD thesis completed in 2004/5. This showed an effectiveness of HP of 90.4% (95% CI 87.6% - 93.2%)[22].

4. Massive regional and national interventions. Two examples are current: **Firstly,** the Finlay Institute in Cuba, a W.H.O. registered vaccine manufacturer, homeopathically immunised the

population of the three worst hit provinces during a 2007 outbreak of leptospirosis, and again in 2008 following severe hurricanes in both years (hurricanes cause increased levels of standing water through which the bacteria is carried). Over 2.2 million people were protected homeopathically with unambiguous success.

Based on this result, the Cuban government instructed the Finlay Institute to homeopathically immunise the entire country over 12 months of age against swine flu during the 2009/10 scare. Over 9.8 million people were immunised and only a handful of cases of swine flu were recorded. In addition, the incidence of pneumococcal disease, which was also covered in the immunisation intervention, declined during that period.

During my third visit to the Finlay Institute in Cuba in March 2012 to collect data, I witnessed the release of their latest homeopathic immunisation against Dengue Fever, and saw data on their Hepatitis A immunisation programs using HP.

Secondly, the provincial government of Andhra Pradesh province in India (population around 97 million) authorised the use of HP against Japanese Encephalitis in 1999, 2000, and 2001. Around 20 million children were immunised. The intervention saw the complete elimination of deaths from JE in Andhra Pradesh by 2003, while levels remained unchanged in the surrounding provinces which did not use HP. These interventions have been documented and published[23].

Whilst orthodox authorities will dismiss the evidence noted above, representatives should be asked if they have indeed studied this material, especially the massive HP interventions conducted by orthodox scientists and medical doctors employed by Government institutions. If they have not, then their comments are no more than being uninformed allegations rather than careful scientific analysis. The mechanism of action of HP may not be understood in orthodox medical terms, but its effectiveness can be observed and measured. This was done with, for example, Asprin which was used for decades because its effectiveness was known, even though its mechanism of action was not known.

Suggestions for parents who use HP

If you use HP and need to discuss your choice with a medical professional or family or friends then I can offer the following suggestions:

1. Start with a point of agreement. Let others know that you fully support immunisation against potentially serious diseases. Make it clear to them that you are choosing to immunise your children – it's just that you are using a method that is different to what they are recommending or using.

2. If they say that HP is worthless and that there is "nothing there", or that there is no evidence, then politely remind them that HP has been used for as many years as vaccination (over 200), and that there is considerable evidence which they appear not to be aware of, but which has been published in books and peer reviewed professional journals.

3. If they say that they have studied the entire evidence base of HP (highly unlikely) and still claim that it is of no value then you are probably best to agree to disagree. If you are confident in your facts then you could point out that the credibility of the evidence base of pharmaceutical medicine (including vaccines) has been deeply compromised by the corrupting influence of Big Pharma, and that this has been demonstrated in publications by highly credible orthodox professionals. Also, that no large long-term safety studies of vaccines have been published.

4. If the person simply refuses to listen openly to what you are saying then it is unlikely that continuing with the discussion will produce anything other than anger or distress. You have said all you can and it is time to move on.

Chapter 4: Drawing the Evidence into a Conclusion

The following conclusions follow from the above analysis:

(i) Vaccination offers a level of protection against targeted infectious diseases, but is not a risk-free procedure.

(ii) Evidence supporting long-term vaccine safety is incomplete and at the best is only suggestive of safety.

(iii) Studies exist suggesting there is a possibility of significant long-term damage from vaccines.

(iv) There is a time-tested and proven alternative to vaccination. On the basis of evidence, HP provides a level of protection against infectious diseases that appears to be comparable to vaccination and is non-toxic.

So it is very reasonable for intelligent and questioning parents to consider whether their child should be homeopathically immunised as an option to vaccination.

Evidence demonstrates that this will offer the child a level of protection that is similar to vaccination but with zero risk of toxic damage.

You do have choices!!

Chapter 5: Practical Immunisation Options

HP can be used for both short-term and long-term prevention of targeted infectious diseases.

Short-term prevention

We use lower potencies given more frequently when trying to combat infectious diseases that are active in the community, or which are active in countries to which we are planning to travel.

My programs generally use 200C potencies every fortnight. When travelling, I recommend starting preventative treatment 1 month before leaving, and continue whilst away. If a disease appears in a child's school for example, I would suggest a fortnightly dose for 4-6 weeks then reassess the situation.

If exposure is definite and intense, then weekly or even twice-weekly doses can be given.

Long-term prevention

My 6 year HP program for long-term prevention commences at 1 month of age and gives a monthly dose of a different remedy for 10 months and then a different dose every 3-4 months after that. The instructions tell parents what to do if they start late, or have to delay the program due to illness, or if they wish to add in other remedies.

My long-term program for Australian conditions is broken into two parts:

(i) **The Main Program** – remedies cover Whooping cough, Pneumococcal disease, Hib (haemophilus influenza B), Meningococcal disease and Tetanus.

(ii) **The Supplementary Program** – remedies cover Polio, Hepatitis B, Rota Virus, Measles, Influenza and Tetanus wounds.

However a different program may be applicable in different countries where diseases such as Japanese Encephalitis, Diphtheria or Dengue Fever may be active, unlike in Australia.

Both the short term and long term programs are flexible. The aim is to cover what is needed in a structured and effective manner.

Remember always that no system of disease prevention is 100% effective, and this applies to HP as well as to vaccination. There is always risk in life, but we are looking at ways to minimise harm from both potentially serious infectious diseases as well as from the method of prevention used.

There is no point giving a safe treatment if it is ineffective. Alternatively, there is no point giving an effective treatment if it can cause serious harm to many recipients. There is no perfect immunisation option, neither vaccination, or HP, or just making your child as healthy as possible.

But HP does offer you an evidence-based middle path where you are providing a significant level of protection without the risk of toxic damage.

Balance in all things!!

Conclusions

I have been personally involved in this issue for 35 years, firstly as a parent of a vaccine damaged child, and then as a homeopathic practitioner discovering that the founder of homeopathy first used "similar" remedies to prevent targeted infectious diseases in 1798, and then more recently to become an active researcher collecting data from around the world to help build the evidence base of HP.

Every week I deal with concerned parents, many of whom have been verbally abused by doctors, or family members, or members of the public, because they have dared to question the "official" position regarding vaccination. And every week I deal with parents of vaccine damaged children.

I have patients who have chosen, after careful research, to vaccinate their children. They have my full support, as do parents who choose to use HP and parents who choose to use neither method of disease prevention.

And so they should – any parents who have taken the time to research and carefully consider all options, and then make an informed decision, deserve the full support of medical professionals as well as health officials and politicians. Such support is sadly lacking in Australia, as well as in other countries whose health systems are dominated by Big Pharma.

But as a parent you can do no more than your best. Collect as much balanced information as you can, make what you see to be the best possible decision, and then own it. Take comfort in the knowledge that you are doing more than most do, and that you acting as a loving and caring parent.

This little booklet is for, and is dedicated to, parents who care.

Resources:

Over the years I have developed a range of resources for parents and practitioners of any modality to use. They include books and web based courses (in English) available from www.homstudy.net.

Books

For Parents

Vaccination & Homoeoprophylaxis?A Review of Risks and Alternatives. 7th ed. 2010.
The 7th edition has been restructured, with extensive new reference material in all sections. A new Section on the use of HP in Cuba involving millions of people has been added, with never before released data. Examines the risks and benefits of vaccination, with the most authoritative discussion of the homoeopathic alternative available. Includes details of Isaac's research over 25 years, including his Doctoral studies, and the history of the homoeopathic alternative. The outstanding reference book for both parents and practitioners researching this contentious topic. 160x225, 440 pages.

Vaccine Damaged Children: Treatment, Prevention, Reasons. (revised 2010).
This book examines what is possibly the most unrecognised public health problem in our community; the long-term impact of vaccination on the general health of children and adults. The book provides data which shows that vaccines cause damage, and details the findings of Isaac's new "reverse" research quantifying the symptoms caused by vaccines. Homoeopathic treatment of vaccine damage is described, including cases of both long and short term treatment are shown. This is a book for practitioners of all modalities, but especially homoeopaths. It is also a book for parents, and an Appendix introducing homoeopathic method is provided. 160x225. 148 pages.

For Practitioners

The Complete Practitioner's Manual of Homœoprophylaxis: A Practical Handbook of Homeopathic Immunisation. 2012.
This book is deliberately aimed at practitioners and students, and is intended to provide a complete, practical, "how-to" guide to implement both short-term and long-term HP programs, although it may help those parents who want to deeply investigate the topic. It contains pages of answers to the most commonly asked questions by parents who are using an HP program,

or considering use. Practical knowledge accumulated over 30 years is presented. As well, the Manual contains the very latest international research on the evidentiary base of HP, including interventions from India and Cuba. It responds to all challenges to HP, and discusses the philosophical basis of HP. 220 pages.

Web based courses

The courses use the latest Camtasia technology where participants log onto a web site, are provided with full powerpoint slides as well as a transcription of the lecture, and see video capture of Isaac talking to the slides, similar to a live presentation. As well, participants can email any questions they may have to the site, and these will be answered by Isaac. The material is available to be accessed at any time, and people are not required to be online at prescribed times as with live webinars. Educationally, it is the best of all options.

For parents:
Immunisation Options: A course for parents who care
As the title says, this course is designed for parents who genuinely care about the health of their children, and who are prepared to take the time to carefully examine health options, and not just rely on being directed by health authorities.
This course faces one of the most difficult of all health decisions that most new parents have to face – how best to protect their child against potentially serious infectious diseases? The reason why it is a difficult decision is firstly because there is no perfect option available, and secondly because there is a considerable amount of misinformation about immunisation options both from orthodox health authorities and from some opponents of vaccination.

This course is not "anti" anything; it is pro-facts, it is pro-informed choice, and it believes that most parents have the intelligence to make sound decisions if they are given reliable and truthful information.

So the objectives of this course are as follows:
1. To provide balanced, well researched, factual information about infectious diseases and alternative methods of disease prevention (immunisation).
2. To empower parents to act with confidence in whatever immunisation decision they make.
3. To provide parents with practical skills to act on the decisions they make.
The course is divided into the following 4 weekly sessions, with a final brief Session 5:

For Practitioners:
The Complete Practitioners Course in Homœoprophylaxis
The aim of the course is to offer homœoprophylaxis (HP) as a tool for any practitioner who has patients/clients who are considering/researching or requesting an alternative to conventional vaccination - A complete packaged solution to offer homœoprophylaxis effectively and confidently.
The following benefits or outcomes for practitioners are expected: -
1) Complete explanation of the HP protocols for both short-term and long-term protection from start to finish in a balanced, integrative way.
2) Confidence in offering the service safely and legally, with templates and paperwork which Isaac personally uses.
3) Management strategies for reactions or other issues which may arise during implementation of HP schedules, with examples from commonly encountered situations in Isaac's practice.
4) How to talk with parents and GP's, with the most common FAQ's Isaac has encountered in his career.
5) Complete supportive evidence, with studies on homœoprophylaxis from 1798 to 2012.
6) Case examples from Isaac's own practice.
7) One on One contact with Isaac throughout the course so that every question you have on the topic can be answered by Isaac.
There are 12 sessions running at least 30 minutes.

Details of these and other resources available at www.homstudy.net

References:

[1] An example occurred in May 2013 in Australia when the public broadcaster SBS ran a program "Jabbed". Far from being a balanced look at the vaccination debate, it presented a heavily biased view which even objective supporters of vaccination saw as lacking objectivity.

[2] NVICP Compensation Data, 2012. **National Vaccine Injury Compensation Program.** US Department of Health and Human Resources. HRSA – Health Resources and Services Administration. http://www.hrsa.gov/vaccinecompensation/data.html.

[3] VAERS

[4] Golden I. *The Complete Practitioners Manual of Homoeoprophylaxis*. Isaac Golden Publications, Gisborne, Australia. 2012.

[5] Stamatakis E, Weiler R, Ioannidis JPA. Undue industry influences that distort healthcare research, strategy, expenditure and practice: a review. *Eur J Clin Invest* 2013; **43**(5): 469–475.

[6] Press release, Cambridge, MA, September 30, 2013. JLME Issue on Institutional Corruption and the Pharmaceutical Industry. A special issue of the Journal of Law Medicine and Ethics. http://www.ethics.harvard.edu/lab/featured/325-jlme-symposium?layout=default#stayinformed.

[7] Golden I. Medical Evidence, Non-Science and Homoeopathy. *Similia*. June 2014; **26**(1):9-14.

[8] NVICP Compensation Data, 2014. **National Vaccine Injury Compensation Program.** US Department of Health and Human Resources. HRSA – Health Resources and Services Administration - Statistics. http://www.hrsa.gov/vaccinecompensation/statisticsreports.html#Stats (accessed 25.1.15).

[9] Australian Academy of Science. *The Science of Immunisation: Questions and Answers*. Australian Academy of Science, November, 2012. Page 12.

[10] Hewitson L, et al, Influence of pediatric vaccines on amygdala growth and opiod ligand binding in rhesus macaque infants: A pilot study. Acta Neurobiol Ezp. 2010; **70**: 147-164.

[11] Odent M. (1994) Long-term effects of early vaccinations. *Primal Health Research*. Vol. 2, No. 1. Pages 3 – 7.

[12] Golden I. (2010) *Vaccination & Homoeoprophylaxis? A Review of Risks and Alternatives*. 7th edition. Isaac Golden Publications, Gisborne, Victoria. Page 164.

[13] Generation Rescue. (2007) *Cal-Oregan vaccinated v's unvaccinated survey*. http://drtenpenny.com/vaccinated_vs_unvaccinated_survey.aspx

[14] Bachmair A (2012) State of health of unvaccinated children. www.vaccineinjury.info/

[15] Australian Academy of Science. *The Science of Immunisation: Questions and Answers.* Australian Academy of Science, November, 2012. Page 12, Box 8.

[16] IOM (Institute of Medicine). 2012. *Adverse effects of vaccines: Evidence and causality.* Washington, DC: The National Academies Press.

[17] Parker SK et al, Thimerosal-Containing Vaccines and Ustistic Spectrum Disorder: A Critical Review of Published Original Data. Pediatrics. 3/9/2004. 3/9/2004; **114**(3):793-804.

[18] Trelka JA, Hooker BS (2004) More on Madsen's Analysis. Correspondence. *J Am Physicians and Surgeons.* Vol. 9, No. 4. P.101.

[19] Email 13/11/2002 from M.B. Lauristen to P Thorsen and K.M. Madsen. Subject : Manuscript about Thimerosal and autism.

[20] Miller NZ, Goldman GS. Infant mortality rates regressed against number of vaccine doses routinely given: Is there a biochemical or synergistic toxicity? *Human and Experimental Toxicology.* **30**(0) 1420-1428.

[21] 65,826 people from 0 to 20 years of age in Blumenau, Brazil were given the homoeopathic remedy Meningococcinum 30c. Another 23,539 people in the area did not receive the remedy. The rates of protection found in the group using HP were **95%** in six months and **91%** in 12 months.

The authors noted that their use of Meningococcinum was not new and cited 12 references to its use from 1966 to 1996. Mroninski C, Adriano E, Mattos G. Meningococcinum: Its protective effect against meningococcal disease. *Homoeopathic Links* Winter, 2001; **14**(4):230-4

[22] Golden I (2010) *Vaccination & Homoeoprophylaxis? A Review of Risks and Alternatives.* Isaac Golden Publications, Gisborne, Australia. 7th edition.

[23] Golden I. (2012) *The Complete Practitioners Manual of Homoeoprophylaxis: A Practical Handbook of Homeopathic Immunisation.* Isaac Golden Publications, Gisborne. Chapter 5.

Printed in Great Britain
by Amazon